A
PRAYER
FOR
CHARLIE

An inspiring, encouraging, life-changing prayer
for those who are HIV positive or have a
sexually transmitted disease

KAREN RAE RUTTY

Copyright © 2018

Author Name: Karen Rae Rutty

ISBN-10: 1721275053

ISBN-13: 978-1721275052

DEDICATION

We all know someone who may have been sick and then died, be it from natural causes, an infectious disease, a deficiency disease, genetic disease, hereditary, or non- hereditary disease, physiological disease, or a sexually transmitted disease.

The pain of losing a loved one can sometimes leave us wondering what we could have done differently to make their lives better.

It is for this reason that I write and dedicate this

book.

I dedicate this book of prayer to all those

who have felt the pain of losing a loved one

through one of the above mentioned.

Additionally, the purpose of writing this

book of prayer is to bring awareness, and to

plead to those who have a sexually transmitted

disease to be more aware and alert of their

illness, and to be cautious of their actions, and

not transmit the disease to others.

I pray you will do all you can to have more

consideration of your friends, family members,

or those with whom you may come in contact with.

Your awareness and consideration will prevent you from giving or spreading the disease intentionally or unintentionally.

This plea is especially for those who may be infected with STD diseases. We love you, and will do all we can to help you, however, we ask that you also love yourself and those with whom you may have sexual relations with.

A Special Dedication to my niece, Rose Thompson

This is a special dedication for my niece, Rose Thompson who passed away on August 9, 2018. After being diagnosed with leukemia in July 2018, Rose passed away on her 56th birthday, August 9, 2018.

Rose, in death your faith was expressed profoundly, thus making our faith profoundly expressed. My beautiful niece…

My beautiful niece, Rose Thompson, I am clinging to my faith in the son of God this morning. "He (Jesus) was a man of sorrows and acquainted with grief" (Isaiah 53:3). I was acquainted with sorrow and grief when I got the news that you transitioned home to glory on your 56th Birthday.

Yesterday, I woke up knowing it was your birthday and believing you will be here with us, but our Heavenly Father and you had other plans. I am reminded of how Jesus, in the book of John 11:35 wept for his friend Lazarus. Rose, I am weeping because you meant so much to me and even though I know you're in a better place it doesn't make things any easier.

Rose, who will remind me on Facebook that "that's my aunty and I am older than her?" You always had so much love and respect for me. Sometimes when you would call me and ask me about Christian books to buy or even scriptures you didn't understand, I would be so amazed by your child-like faith. You were such a sincere, loving, thoughtful person, and kindness was your portion.

Rose, even if I cried a river, Psalm 56:8 told me God would collect every one of my tears. See Rose, words are few right now, but God can articulate my tears and express to you how I am really feeling.

You can rest now my niece. Visiting you in the hospital the last four weeks was heartbreaking for me. Rose, I am sure you are enjoying your new "Place", and I can just see the smile on your face. I find comfort in the truth. Jesus did you well with the "Place" he prepared for you. According to John 14:2b-3 (NIV)," If I go and prepare a place for you, I will come again and receive you to Myself, that where I am, there you may be also."

To my Family and Damarli

Brothers and sisters, we do not want you to be uninformed about those who sleep in death... "... so that you do not grieve like the rest of mankind, who have no hope. For we believe that Jesus died and rose again, and so we believe that God will bring with Jesus those who have fallen asleep in him." (1 Thessalonians 4:13-14, NIV)

I am confident in this, that Rose is alive in Him. Paul said in 1 Corinthians 15:19, " "If we have only hoped in Christ in this life, we are of all men most pitiable."

We know Rose had put her trust in Christ; "...

and to be present with the Lord."

(2 Corinthians 5:8 NKJV)

Rose's portion is paradise" (Luke 23:43

NIV) "... is the death of his faithful servants."

(Psalm 116:15 NIV). Rose has now put on her

new immortal body. I am praising God for his

faithfulness even in the midst of my sorrow.

The scripture give assurance that she is alive

and well. And so now Rose speaks... "and this

mortal has put on immortality, then shall be

brought to pass the saying what is written:

'Death is swallowed up in victory.' 'O Death,

where is your sting? O Hades, where is your victory?'" (1 Corinthians 15:54-55 NIV)

I believe Jesus has made everything new for Rose and she is blessed forever. Rose is seated in heavenly places in Christ Jesus. For the old order of things has passed away. He who was seated on the throne said, 'I am making everything new!'" (Revelation 21:4-5 NIV) So family, "Weeping may endure for a night, but joy comes in the morning." (Psalm 30:5)

ACKNOWLEDGMENTS

First, I would like to acknowledge, and make
mention of some key people in my life. To all
my family members who have transitioned
home to glory due to natural causes, cancer,
heart attack, or any other deadly diseases, this is
for you.

Special thanks to my wonderful husband,
Pastor Andrew Rutty, thank you for being my

greatest supporter, you who always support me.

To my beautiful daughter, Sekeyia, my
handsome son, Zephaniah, and my lovely
granddaughter, Cataleya, you all mean the world
to me.

To: Charlie
From: Karen Rae Rutty
Subject: A Prayer for you

Dear Charlie:

The day when I heard of your story I was moved to pray for you. As a Pastor, one who has a heart for God's sheep, it is my duty to pray for others, instead of judge them.

"For all have sinned and fall short of the glory of God, being justified freely by His grace through the redemption that is in Christ Jesus, whom God set forth as a propitiation by His

Blood, through faith, to demonstrate His righteousness, because in His forbearance God had passed over the sins that were previously committed, to demonstrate at the present time His righteousness, that He might be just, and the justifier of the one who has faith in Jesus" (Romans 3:21-26).

My sincere desire and prayer is that you would find peace in Jesus as I have through this text.

Charlie, there are many people who will have their own opinion about the fact that you have been infected with the HIV virus. But, I want you to know that I am not persuaded or moved by the judgmental attitude of others.

This morning, as I sit in my home in the presence of the Almighty God who loves you, despite of it all, I am moved to pray for you.

Charlie, others will point their fingers and choose to turn their backs on you, but they cannot point their fingers at you without pointing back at themselves. They too have sinned and fall short of the glory of God.

You see, God knew beforehand, that you and I would sin and fall short of His glory, and because He loves us with an everlasting love, He have made a declaration "JUSTIFICATION BY GRACE".

The Lord wanted to remind you and the rest of the world, this day, that you have been redeemed by the blood of Jesus that was shed on Calvary.

Charlie, what Paul was saying to those of us who put our faith in Christ Jesus, is that, we are justified by His grace and Christ was set forth as a propitiation, and to demonstrate His righteousness in us who believed.

For every sin we committed against God, Christ exchanged our sins and gave us God's love. God loves you Charlie. The Word of God, in St. John 3:16 declares "For God so loved the world that He gave His only begotten Son, that whosoever believe upon Him should not perish but have everlasting life. For God did not send His Son into the world to condemn the world, but that the world through Him might be saved."

I pray, and declare God's love over your life, today. I Pray that you accept and receive his love, knowing that he died to give you eternal life.

Charlie, hold your chin up. God loves you with an everlasting love. HIV, cancer, or other diseases cannot separate you from the love of God. The Bible declares, "What shall we say to these things?

The contraction of HIV, the lawsuits, the opinions of people, the lies, and the hates that sprout out of the people who you thought had your back, the greed, and inconsideration of insensitive people may have caused you some pain. Charlie, the scripture says, "If God is for us, who can be against us?".

Charlie, God is for you, despite of it all, He loves you. You might be wondering how I know God is for you. I have experienced God's love in my own life. The Bible also tells us that "He who did not spare His own Son, but delivered Him up for us all, how shall He not with Him also freely give us all things? (Romans 8:33).

So, today, Charlie, I pray healing in your life. I ask Jesus to heal your broken-heart, heal your soul, heal your emotions, heal your mind, heal your body, and heal those who have hurt you, and heal those you have hurt.

The text continues in verse 33 of Romans 8, "Who shall bring a charge against God's elect? It is God who justifies. Who is he who condemns? It's Christ who died, and furthermore is also raised, who is even at the right hand of God, who also makes intercession for us. So, you see, Charlie, I pronounce you, by the blood of Jesus, "not guilty".

Who shall separate us from the love of Christ? Shall tribulation, or distress, or persecution, or famine, or nakedness, or peril, or sword? As it is written: "For your sake we are killed all day long; we are counted as sheep for the slaughter."

Yet in all these things, Charlie, you are more than a conqueror through Him who loves you. Charlie, I am persuaded that neither death nor life, nor angels, nor principalities nor powers, nor things present, nor things to come, nor height nor depth, nor any other created things, shall be able to separate you from the love of God which is in Christ Jesus our Lord.

I really wanted to just let you know I have received and accepted the love of God into my heart, and freely He gave His love to me. I wanted to freely share it with you, hoping you accept him into your heart as well. Matthew

10:8 declared, "Heal the sick, raise the dead, cleanse the lepers, and cast out demons: freely ye received, freely give"

JESUS LOVES YOU CHARLIE. YES, HE DOES!

I AM SURE OF IT!

This is my prayer for you: I pray healing and forgiveness for you.

THE PRAYER:

With the love of Christ in my heart, and in his name, I say this prayer for you, Charlie.

Father, in the name of Jesus Christ, I come to you in prayer asking you to cover Charlie under the precious blood of Jesus.

Lord, I know the real enemy behind his life is the devil, so I bind the hands of the devil, I render Satan powerless and ineffective in Jesus name.

I release the fire of God to burn out every forces of darkness in Charlie's life. I speak to every mountain and pray that every mountain in his life crumble and die in the name of Jesus.

I cast out wandering spirits, and the spirit of addiction. I cast them out in the name of Jesus. I now release the anointing of God in Charlie's life. Anoint him from the crown of his head to the sole of his feet. Lord I thank you. I give you praise, for when You created Charlie, You knew the thoughts and the plans You have for him. They are plans to do good and not evil. You gave him a hope and a future.

SCRIPTURE REFERENCE

The scripture says "For I know the thoughts I think towards you, saith Jehovah, thoughts of peace and not of evil, to give you hope in your latter end. And ye shall call upon me, and ye shall go and pray unto me, and I will hearken unto you. And ye shall seek me, and find me, when ye shall search for me with all your heart. And I will be found of you, saith Jehovah, and I will turn again your captivity, and I will gather you from all the nations, and from all the places whither I have driven you, saith

Jehovah; and I will bring you again unto the place

whence I caused you to be carried away captive.”

(Jeremiah 29:12-14 ASV)

THE PRAYER: You Pray

Now, Charlie, please say this prayer.

Father, in the name of Jesus, I (Put your name here) ______________________________________

confess that I have sinned against heaven and I ask you to forgive me of all my sins. I receive Jesus into my heart today to be my Lord and savior of my life. In Jesus name.

Amen!

Welcome to the Kingdom of God, where there is no judging, just loving!

Dear Reader,

It is not a coincidence that you happen to be reading this prayer that is dedicated to someone who have been infected with HIV or has a sexual transmitted disease.

Whether you are the one who is infected, or you know someone who have been infected with this sexually transmitted disease, I want you to know this that God before time has forgiven you and has turned your captivity around.

The scripture declares in Psalm 103:12-13, that "How far has the Lord taken our sins from us? Further than the distance from the east to the west. As a Father has compassion on His son, so the Lord has compassion on those who fears Him. For He knows what we are made of, remembering that we are dust".

Put your trust in the Lord. His desire is to heal you and make you whole. He wants to bring you back in right standing with him.

God wants to reconcile you to himself. He has made provision for healing through Jesus Christ. If you have been infected with STD, I want to encourage you to make a change in your life today. I exhort you today. Make a change and turn your life around.

I want you to know that Jesus wants to heal you. He wants to set you free. I plead to you to please accept Jesus Christ as your Lord and savior today. Now is the day of salvation. Now is the appointed time for you to be set free.

I pray you will be healed and delivered in Jesus name. Amen!

GOD BLESS YOU!

BE HEALED!

BE DELIVERED!

BE FREE!

BE SAVED!
In Jesus' name, Amen

www.ingramcontent.com/pod-product-compliance
Lightning Source LLC
Chambersburg PA
CBHW070104260726
48658CB00002B/985